THE ESSENTIAL HANDBOOK TO INTERMITTENT FASTING

HOW TO DECIDE IF INTERMITTENT FASTING IS RIGHT FOR YOU INCLUDING TYPES OF FASTS AND TIPS FOR SUCCESS

BY

EVELYN CARMICHAEL

Copyright © 2019

Evelyn Carmichael

TABLE OF CONTENTS

Evelyn Carmichael

LEGAL NOTES

Evelyn Carmichael

INTRODUCTION

The Intermittent Fasting Plan has been getting a lot of buzz of late as it soars in popularity due to the effectiveness as a weight loss tool. Recently, this fasting plan has been retooled from a 24 hour fast to some more popular 16/8 and 5:2 Fasting cycles. This handbook explains the differences between the different fasting plans for you to see if any would fit into your lifestyle.

This book also discusses the science behind why Intermittent Fasting works, the benefits and potential risks of fasting as well as tips to be successful.

Evelyn Carmichael

CHAPTER 1. WHAT IS INTERMITTENT FASTING?

Intermittent Fasting is the pattern of cycles between eating and fasting. It is not a diet per say, but rather a schedule of eating. This can be done through a variety of methods with the most popular being the 24 hour, 16/8 or 5:2 cycles.   This plan has gained headlines of late due to the success people have had with weight loss.

While fasting has been practiced since at least 5BC when Hippocrates famously recommended the absence of food and drink for certain medical conditions, there have not been very many studies looking at the longevity of fasting. However, a recent review of over 40 Intermittent Fasting studies on humans did see some promising effects for weight loss. With an average time span of 10 weeks, the typical weight loss was 7-11 pounds. The methods of Intermittent Fasting and participants differed considerably, and more studies are needed to show if there is a difference between different types of fasting for persons with certain characteristics. Studies replicated with humans have shown the same but no more so than any other diet plan. Many researchers have surmised that some individuals have not had success because traditional fasting can be hard for some people. Not eating for long periods of time can make you irritable and hungry.   However, many studies of late have looked at specific Intermittent Fasting cycles. Studies have shown greater success with not only on how long you stick with this schedule of eating but also how your body responds to it.

The Science Behind Intermittent Fasting

There's a lot of information out there about Intermittent Fasting. However, the information you're likely to come across might not always explain the science behind it. This is a real shame as If you want to really harness the power of Intermittent Fasting you need to fully understand how it works. Understanding Intermittent Fasting can also help you decide which fasting plan would work best for you to be successful.

Some recent scientific studies have shown that the timing is key as it can help you to make your Intermittent Fasting much more effective.

When we eat the food that we consume is broken down by some enzymes that live in our gut. After a while, the food is turned into molecules that enter our bloodstream. The carbohydrates we consume are broken down into sugars. These sugars are used by our cells as they contain energy. If our cells do not use the carbohydrates, they are stored in our fat cells. However, when we consume sugar it is broken down and it is sent to our cells within insulin. Insulin moves the sugar to the fat cells where it stays.

If we don't have a snack in between meals our insulin levels will go down. It is then up to our fat cells to ensure we have enough energy to carry on. They do this by releasing any sugar that has been stored in our cells. If you were to continue to let your insulin levels, go down you will lose weight.

The idea surrounding Intermittent Fasting is that it allows the levels of insulin do go down so far that we eventually burn off all of our fat.

Intermittent Fasting does not have to be hard

While some people undoubtedly find it hard to fast it does not have to be. Studies have shown that those who eat less each day and those who partake in Intermittent Fasting tend to lose the same amount of weight. However, some people struggled on the days that they fasted. The trick here is to make the whole fasting process so much easier. Those who find it hard to eat less every day might benefit from Intermittent Fasting if they know how to get the most out of it.

Intermittent Fasting Cycles

Intermittent Fasting refers to a cycle of eating that includes some periods of fasting. Fasting can last from 12 to 36 hours. Those who have already participated in Intermittent Fasting have reported better weight management and weight loss.

Research has also shown that Intermittent Fasting can:

- Improve your health

- Reduce your risk of some chronic conditions

- Improve brain health

As you can see, there are some clear benefits to embarking on intermittent fasting. If you struggle to reduce your calorific content day-to-day you might find Intermittent Fasting is beneficial. Many people do find it easier to refrain from eating for 24-36 hours than attempting to cut down on what they eat. If you have ever participated in a fast in the past this plan may sound familiar. Determining the schedule of the fast is the first hurdle in success for this plan.

Lowering Insulin Levels

A recent study carried out by the University of Alabama conducted a restricted feeding study. This study involved two groups of obese men. The first group was only allowed to eat between 7 am and 3 pm. The second group of men was only allowed to eat between 7 am and 7 pm. Each of the groups had their meals during the set hours. They were not allowed to consume any food after the set hours.

Both groups of men did not lose or gain any weight after a period of 5 weeks. However, those who were in the 7 am to 3 pm group had lower insulin levels. In addition to this, their blood pressure was also slightly lower. Both group's appetites were significantly decreased.

What this means is that if you change when you eat your meals your metabolism is likely to benefit from it. This study just goes to show that there is indeed some benefit behind changing your eating patterns and looking carefully at the time of day you choose to restrict your feeding. Timing your eating window to avoid eating and then going right to bed. While the study only shows a five-week window, it is of note that you should also pay attention to what and how much you are eating during the non-fasting times.

The study did not change what the men ate, merely when they ate. A benefit of lower insulin levels was seen in the five week period. Watching what you eat and what hours you eat may be more beneficial than just the timing of the fasting hours alone.

Evelyn Carmichael

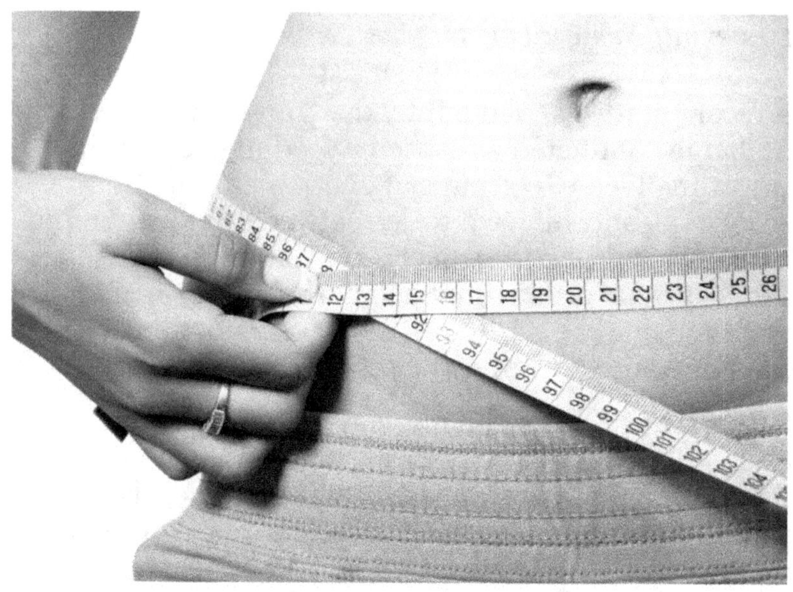

Benefits of Fasting

Boosts Weight Loss
Increases Energy
Lowers Bad Cholesterol
Reduces Insulin Resistance
Generate Antioxidants
Boost Metabolism
Increase Cellular Repair
Lower Waist Circumference
Reduce Inflammation
Increases Brain and Heart Health

Risks

While there are definite benefits to fasting, there are also some risks. Especially when introducing fasting to your lifestyle, there can be hunger, muscle aches, fatigue, dizziness, and irritability to name a few. However, once your body is used to the fast cycle, most of these negative attributes lessen or go away completely. In fact, most people find they eat less during the non-fast periods and have more energy while fasting.

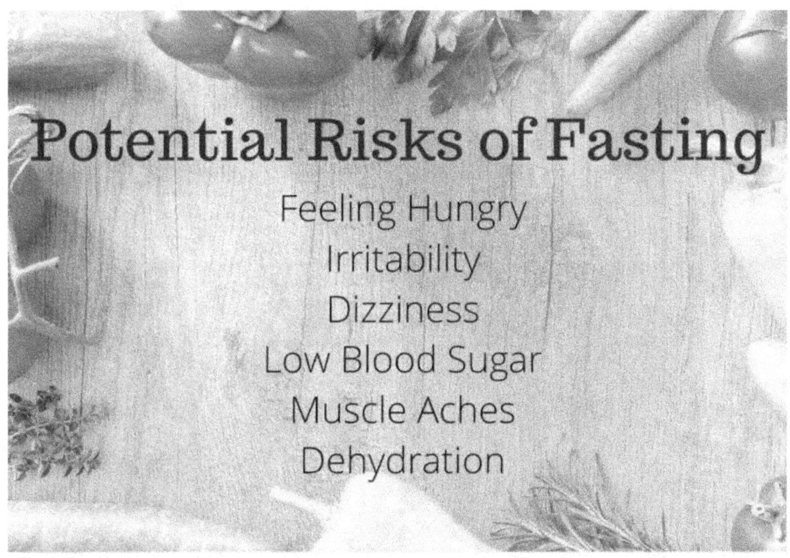

Prolonged fasting can present more significant risks. Prolonged fasting can last three days up to a month and has been associated with kidney and liver issues, irregular heartbeats, muscle breakdown, and vitamin and mineral deficiencies.   Prolonged fasting can be potentially dangerous for your body.

You should consult your physician before undergoing any type of dietary change. Likewise, having certain medical conditions such as diabetes, pregnancy, or adolescents should not participate in Intermittent Fasting.

Next, we will look at three popular Intermittent Fasting plans to see which one might fit with your lifestyle.

The Essential Handbook to Intermittent Fasting

CHAPTER 2. THE 24-HOUR FAST

Intermittent fasting can consist of a 24 hour fast which is a very popular way to control your weight. This fast basically means that you do not eat anything for 24 hours. While refraining from your regular eating schedule can be quite hard for some individuals, the rewards can be quite striking. At the end of the 24 hours, you would eat a meal of normal size.

You can do more than one 24 hours fast a week should you wish to. Some people do as many as 3 fasts a week. However, you should do no more than 3 fasts as research has shown this is not effective for overall body health.

THE 24-HOUR WATER FAST

The 24-Hour water fast consists of refraining from eating or drinking anything apart from water. The 24-Hour water fast has the same benefits as the 24-Hour fast. However, one of the good things about this diet is that drinking water can help to keep you feeling full. This is not to say that you should drink a lot of water, but it can help you to feel less hungry.

When you fast for 24 hours it means you won't have anything to eat for 24 hours. So, if your diet were to start at 10 am on a Tuesday you would not eat until 10 am on the Wednesday.
An average person's body needs from 1,800 to 2,400 calories a day. The body has from 400 to 600 grams of glycogen. This is a type of carbohydrate that is used as energy. A single gram of glycogen provides as much as 4 calories. This means that an average body holds between 1,600 and 3,600 calories.

When you don't eat your body uses the glycogen up, so it has enough energy for the day. When these glycogen stores are used up your body will get energy from the fat your body is storing. When the body enters this stage, which is known as "Ketosis" you're more likely to lose weight.

A 24 hour fast will ensure your body enters ketosis. However, this all depends on how active you are. If you were to exercise on your fasting day you will reach ketosis much earlier than someone who remains sedentary.

THE BENEFITS OF THE 24 HOUR FAST

- KETOSIS

We have already seen that ketosis can help you to lose weight. But did you know that ketones are great for your brain? When you're in a state of ketosis you will have better productivity and attention.

- Autophagy
This is a process whereby cells are recycled. As someone ages their body gains a lot of damaged cells. Some of these cells can lead to serious conditions such as cancer. If you refrain from eating, your body will speed up the cell recycling process. When this occurs, your damaged cells are used for energy before being replaced by new and fully functioning cells.

- Weight loss

One of the most obvious benefits to the 24-hour fast is weight loss. Your body will burn glycogen and any fat that is stored in your body. If you drink water while you're on this diet it will leave the body as urine. Making sure you are well hydrated also aids in digestion when you are in the non-fasting hours.

- Better sugar levels

Your body can control your blood sugar levels by secreting insulin. The older we are the more insulin our bodies need to control the sugar level. This is known as insulin resistance and can cause type 2 diabetes.

When you fast for 24 hours insulin is only minimally to not secreted. This means that you will have improved insulin sensitivity. If you can control your insulin levels over a long period of time with periods of fasting, studies have shown that prediabetes can be reversed or the need for medication to be decreased.

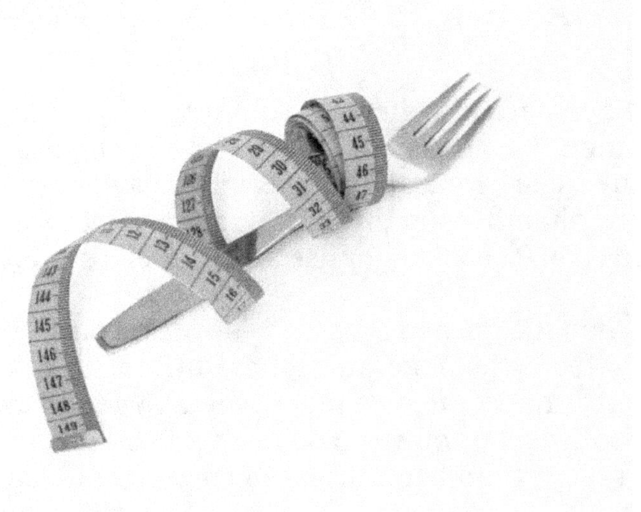

Signs of Ketosis

Decreased Appetite
Weight Loss
Ketosis Breath
Short-Term Fatigue
Decrease in Productiveness
High Energy
Digestive Issues
Muscle Cramps
Headaches
Increased Focus

--

WHAT SHOULD I EAT AND DRINK?

When partaking in the 24-hour fast you should drink water, tea, and coffee. However, you should not add any sugar. You can drink as much as you wish.
You should avoid drinking sugary drinks and eating snacks. Please do not use any artificial sweeteners.

When it comes to breaking your fast you should try to eat foods that contain a lot of nutrients. Try to eat a salad that contains a lot of vegetables. Add fats such as olive oil or butter. You can also add an egg or two. Try to refrain from eating too much seafood or meet.

THE DOWNSIDES OF A 24 HOUR FAST

When you first embark on a 24 hour fast you are likely to feel very hungry. You might even get a bit of indigestion. Do not worry though, these side effects will go away.

You might also feel dizzy or have a headache. However, the more often you fast the less likely you are to experience these side effects.

WHO CAN DO A 24 HOUR FAST?

Anyone who is over the age of 18 and has no pre-existing medical condition can fast. If you are pregnant or breastfeeding, you should refrain from fasting. Those who have a pre-existing medical condition should speak to their doctor first before starting any fasting plan.

CHAPTER 3. OTHER TYPES OF INTERMITTENT FASTING CYCLES

THE 16/8 PLAN VS THE 5:2 PLAN

If you've not tried Intermittent Fasting, chances are you know someone who has. They might have tried Intermittent Fasting so they can lose weight, lower their insulin levels, or simply feel healthier.

While fasting is by no means a new concept, over the last few years there has been a lot of research undertaken. This research has shown that Intermittent Fasting is very beneficial not just for weight loss but for overall health. But which option will you opt for? There are two popular Intermittent Fasting Options, though you can tailor any plan to fit your needs. Will you go for the 16/8 plan or the 5:2 plan? It can be hard to decide which option is better for you or if you should modify to a different plan. The good news is you can find information about these options below:

WHAT IS THE 16/8 PLAN?

The 16/8 diet limits your eating to 8 hours in a day. This does not mean that you should eat for 8 hours, you simply have 8 hours to eat your meals. You would then have 16 hours left to fast each day.

During the 8-hour period, it's recommended that you eat 2 main meals or 3 smaller meals. This helps to control the amount of calories you consume. The 16-hour period where you don't have any food will help your body to kick start your metabolism. This will help to reduce your insulin levels and inflammation.

THE PROS AND CONS OF THE 16/8 PLAN

The 16/8 plan is easy to stick to if you can get through your morning hunger and refrain from eating until 10 am or midday. You can then have 2-3 balanced meals during the remaining 8 hours.

If you eat a balanced diet you can still lose weight. However, you do not need to count your calories as such. Just make sure that your meals are nutritional and filling.

If you have trouble keeping your calorific intake quite low this diet could be an option for you. If you don't have the energy, time, or concentration to manage your food intake on low-calorie days, the 16/8 plan is much more likely to help.

In addition to this, the 16/8 plan is quite easy to follow over a long period of time.

WHAT IS THE 5/2 PLAN?

This is a regime that seems to have caught the attention of the world. This is the 'original' Intermittent Fasting plan. Those who partake in this diet are encouraged to fast for 2 days a week. These days should not follow each other. The 2 'fast' days should consist of you consuming less than 500 or 600 calories a day. The rest of the week you can eat as you normally do.

Research showed that limiting the intake of calories to this extent helped to boost the metabolism, it also helps to sustain weight loss.

THE PROS AND CONS OF THE 5/2 PLAN

The 5/2 plan can be a very effective plan if you can stick to it. However, it's not always very easy to do. Some people really struggle to consume only 500 calories on their fast day. Five hundred calories are equal to a small salad with some fish, one egg and perhaps some coffee with cream.

If you can stick with it, the 5/2 plan can help you to lose weight. However, you will need to be strict with yourself. Some people imagine that they can consume up to 1,000 calories (or two small meals) and reap the same rewards, but this is not the case. You will be less likely to lose quite as much weight if you're eating twice the amount of calories.

If you have a busy life and you tend to be quite active the 5/2 plan might prove to be tough for you. However, it can be ideal for those who don't tend to eat very much until their evening meal where they consume a lot. If they can control how much they eat during their evening meal the plan could work well for them. In addition to this, they will not need to count their calories on the other 5 days.

MODIFICATIONS

There are many different ways you can modify the 16-8 or 5:2 plan to fit your lifestyle. Some people are very successful on a 16:8 during the week coupled with low carbohydrate eating and then on weekends not counting calories or fasting. Others mix the 5:2 with a 16-8 and have just one day of fasting and do a 14 or 15 hour fast the other days. The key is to find what is providing the results that you are looking for and that you can continue to keep it as part of your lifestyle.

BEING CONSISTENT

If you decide to undertake an Intermittent Fasting Plan you should try to be as consistent as you can. There is a lot of evidence the shows fasting occasionally is good for us. This is because it not only helps us to reset our metabolism, but it helps us to feel naturally hungry and eat less overall. Therefore, we are more likely to achieve weight loss.

FASTING THAT WORKS FOR YOU

One of the key aspects of embarking on an Intermittent Fasting Plan is to find a fast that works for you. If you can find a plan that you can stick to you should see significant results in 8 to 12 weeks, though there are the lucky few who see results quickly. Please note, fasting is not a quick-fix solution, it is merely a lifestyle choice that can help to control your weight. You just have to make sure you stick to it so you can reap the rewards.

Evelyn Carmichael

CHAPTER 4. TIPS TO SUCCESSFUL INTERMITTENT CYCLING

Here are a few hints and tips to help ensure success with Intermittent Cycling.

WATER

It is especially important when fasting to keep up your water intake. You need to keep your body hydrated while it is going into ketosis and water is vital for this. If you are getting bored with plain water, it is fine to add a squeeze of lemon or try a sparkling variety.

Evelyn Carmichael

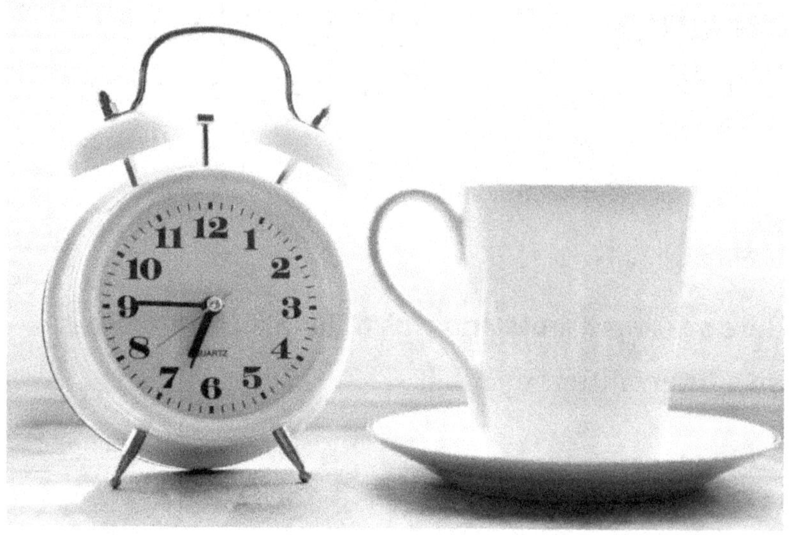

Beverages while Fasting

WATER
Sparkling Water- including Flavored
Black Coffee
Unsweetened Tea
1-2 TBS Apple Cider Vinegar

WHAT CAN I ADD TO MY TEA AND COFFEE?

The general rule is that if you add anything over 50 calories, you are breaking your fast. However, there are some choices better than others.

Stevia does not break down in the body in a way that causes insulin levels to spike. If you decide to add stevia, make sure you are getting the organic variety as there are stevia producers that add sucrose and alcohol sugars.

WHAT IS ALL THE FUSS ABOUT BULLETPROOF COFFEE?

Bulletproof coffee is a branded coffee that starts with a cup of black coffee and you blend in a tablespoon of full fat butter or ghee and a tablespoon of MCT oil. This is a special type of oil where medium-chain level triglycerides from palm kernel oil or coconut oil. This concoction can have 100 to well over 100-250 calories depending how made so people often ask if preparing coffee this way would break their fast. A 16 oz cup of coffee with 1 tablespoon of MCT oil 1 tablespoon of butter has 230 calories. The short answer is yes, technically speaking, anything over 50 calories will break your fast. However, not all 50 calories are the same, and that is where this question becomes more complicated.   Full fat butter (or ghee) as well as MCT oils do not impact insulin levels, so some make the argument that this coffee will make you feel full and not impact your fast.   This coffee may be a good addition if doing a straight ketogenic diet plan, but for fasting, it technically does break your fast. It may be a better alternative as the first "meal" of your eating hours.

The same idea goes toward bone broth. The nutrient rich broth helps replace electrolytes, but technically will break your fast. However, bone broth does not take you out of ketosis.

What Can I Add to My Coffee?

Splash of Heavy Cream

Tablespoon of Unsweetened Almond Milk

Tablespoon of Coconut Milk

WHAT ABOUT OTHER NON-CALORIC DRINKS?

There are two schools of thought on this with differing research. Some stay strict to the rule that it is all about the calories. If you want to add Stevia to iced tea or coffee or have a diet soda that would be fine as you are not adding calories to break your fast. Other research shows that having diet soda triggers sugar cravings and would make it more difficult for you to stay on the fast. Studies have also shown diet soda to negatively affect gut bacteria and insulin secretion.

Stevia does not break down in the body in a way that causes insulin levels to spike. If you decide to add stevia, make sure you are getting the organic variety as there are stevia producers that add sucrose and alcohol sugars.

KEEPING TRACK

As this plan allows some leeway with the number of hours you fast, make sure you are keeping close track of the amount of hours you fast along with your weight to see variances and what will work best for you. There are Intermittent Fasting Logbooks or just a plain calendar would work to write down the number of hours fasted and a weekly weight. If you see inconsistencies in the amount of hours and weight loss, you may want to pay closer attention and log what you are eating in during the non-fasting hours to see if too many carbohydrates are interfering with weight loss. Many individuals combine a pseudo Keto Diet with Intermittent Fasting for optimal weight loss.

MINDSET

When starting the Intermittent Plan, it is very important to think of this as your new schedule of eating. As it is ingrained in most of us from an early age to have meals at set times, you will be embarking on setting your body to a new clock. Don't think of this as a diet. Likewise, don't get discouraged if one day circumstances change so that your fast is changed. Sometimes people eat at different times and just get right back to your pre-determined schedule of eating the following day. You are in control of your schedule and the Intermittent Fasting Plan can be highly effective if you allow for variances and then get right back to it.

CHAPTER 5. REFERENCES

1. Jane L, Atkinson G, Jaime V, Hamilton S, Waller G, Harrison S. Intermittent fasting interventions for the treatment of overweight and obesity in adults aged 18 years and over: a systematic review protocol. JBI Database System Rev Implement Rep. 2015 Oct;13(10):60-8. doi: 10.11124/jbisrir-015-2363.

2. Collier R. Intermittent fasting: the science of going without. *CMAJ*. 2013;185(9): E363–E364. doi:10.1503/cmaj.109-4451

3. Harris L, Hamilton S, Azevedo LB, Olajide J, De Brún C, Waller G, Whittaker V, Sharp T, Lean M, Hankey C, Ells L. Intermittent fasting interventions for treatment of overweight and obesity in adults: a systematic review and meta-analysis., JBI Database System Rev Implement Rep. 2018 Feb;16(2):507-547. doi: 10.11124/JBISRIR-2016-003248.

4. Stockman MC, Thomas D, Burke J, Apovian CM. Intermittent Fasting: Is the Wait Worth the Weight? *Curr Obes Rep*. 2018;7(2):172–185. doi:10.1007/s13679-018-0308-9

5. Wilson RA, Deasy W, Stathis CG, Hayes A, Cooke MB. Intermittent Fasting with or without Exercise Prevents Weight Gain and Improves Lipids in Diet-Induced Obese Mice. *Nutrients*. 2018;10(3):346. Published 2018 Mar 12. doi:10.3390/nu10030346

Read on for an excerpt of Evelyn Carmichael's book *The Essential Handbook to Carb Cycling and the Ketogenic Diet*, now on Amazon.

THE ESSENTIAL HANDBOOK TO CARB CYCLING AND THE KETOGENIC DIET

HOW TO MAKE THE CHANGES NEEDED TO BE SUCCESSFUL WITH CARB CYCLING AND HOW IT RELATES TO THE KETO DIET INCLUDING FREQUENT QUESTIONS, MEAL PLANS, AND SHOPPING LISTS

BY

EVELYN CARMICHAEL

44

INTRODUCTION

If you are considering going on a diet you may have heard of the very popular Ketogenic diet and the derivative Carb Cycling Diet. This diet has found worldwide acclaim thanks to its ability to help people lose weight and keep it off for good. While there are a lot of other diets out there it seems that the Ketogenic diet is a highly effective one that continues to make headlines even today.

Carb Cycling is a variation that you will learn about that take components of the Keto Diet and is modified to fit your lifestyle. This handbook will explain what Keto and Carb Cycling is and how to understand the world of macronutrients so you can successfully count carbs. If you're serious about losing weight and you want a sustainable diet change, the Ketogenic diet could be successful for you.

People who are ultimately successful on the Keto diet has a good understanding of macronutrients. This is discussed a lot in this book, but basically it is a grasp on the building blocks of the food you eat and how it effects your body. Keeping track of your net carbs is vital to success and this book will teach you how to do so at home and when you go out to eat. While some diets are about calorie counting, this is more of an accounting of what the food is made of that you are consuming.

Once you understand the Keto diet, you may want to modify this diet plan to do carb cycling. This handbook will explain what carb cycling is and you will be able to determine which method best fits your lifestyle.
If you are diabetic, pregnant, breastfeeding or you have had your gallbladder removed you will need to make some adjustments that are discussed in this book. This Essential Handbook will tell you how to stick to the Ketogenic diet while ensuring your body gets the nutrients it always needs. As with any type of diet, make sure you consult with your physician before starting.

CHAPTER 1. HOW DOES THE KETOGENIC DIET WORK?

The Ketogenic Diet has been proven to help you lose weight. This diet works by ensuring you limit your intake of carbohydrates so that your body begins to burn fat as opposed to sugar. When your body burns energy it firstly begins to burn any blood sugar (Carbohydrates) that you've eaten. As soon as the sugar has been burned your body will begin to burn stored fat (ketone bodies). This is called ketosis.

When you start eating according to the 'Rules' of the Ketogenic Diet you will start to eat fewer carbohydrates. This means that your body will burn fewer sugars simply because you haven't consumed as many and will, therefore, burn more fat. It is this aspect of the diet that ensures you're are much more likely to lose weight. In other words, you will burn more fat than you'll consume, which is ideal for weight loss.

How long does it take for the body to switch from using blood sugar to ketone bodies?

After just 2-4 days on the Keto Diet, your body will start to make big changes. It will begin to go into ketosis and start using stored fat for energy. For most individuals, this is accomplished by eating 20 to 50 grams of carbohydrates a day.

MACRONUTRIENTS

Macronutrients are the building blocks of your diet and consist of protein, carbohydrates, and fats. Getting your macronutrient ratio right is essential as macronutrients form the base of your diet. Getting your macronutrients right is essential as doing so will help you to lose weight.

MACRONUTRIENTS

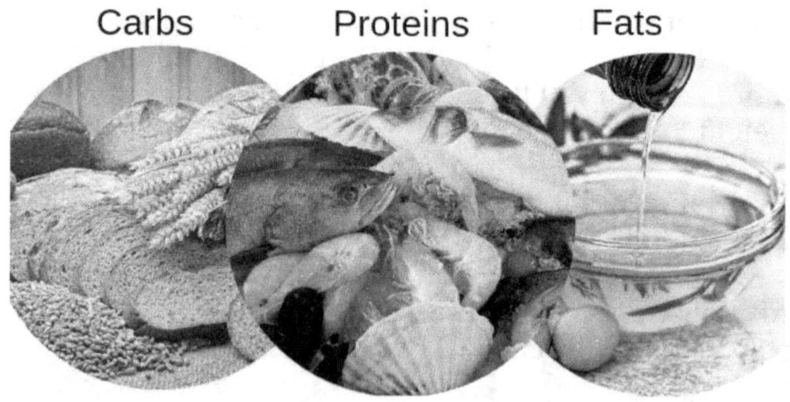

You should ideally get no more than ten percent of your calories from carbohydrates. No more than thirty percent of your calories from protein and no more than 60 percent of your calories from fat. It is essential that you work out where all your calories come from. When you can get the macronutrient ration right you will start to lose weight. This is because the macronutrients will come from many different sources rather than meals that are full of fat and sugar.

HOW DO I KNOW IF I AM IN KETOSIS?

The chart below shows some of the signs of being in ketosis. While some signs are positive, such as losing weight, there are some side effects, such as ketone breath (fruity smelling) that may be found. Also, while the chart shows some more obvious signs, a blood test is the most definitive measure to show ketones in your blood. Blood test results will show .5-3 millimoles of blood ketones per liter. There are at home breath and urine kits available as well.

PROOF?

Due to the popularity of the Ketogenic Diet, there have been many studies examining the effect of the Ketogenic Diet and its effect on weight loss. One of the early studies in 2004 looked at the long- time effects of the diet (24 weeks) and found that not only did Body Mass Index BMI) decrease significantly but bad cholesterol levels (LDL) went down and good cholesterol (HDL) levels went up. Triglyceride levels also decreased significantly. Furthermore, a 2017 study looked at the Ketogenic Diet in Endocrine Disorders and found that there is clinical evidence to support the use of KD in diabetes, obesity, and endocrine disorders.

To find out how if Carb Cycling and the Ketogenic Diet is right for you, please visit https://www.amazon.com/dp/B07Y1311ZK.

Evelyn Carmichael

ABOUT THE AUTHOR

Evelyn Carmichael

Evelyn was in the world of corporate finance before switching her life path after a successful battle with breast cancer. She is a personal life coach, fitness guru, and healthy lifestyle advocate. She has written over 20 healthy living books including the bestselling book The Essential Handbook to Lectin.

Find out more on Facebook or at https://www.amazon.com/Evelyn-Carmichael/e/B01MQYHZLC

Evelyn Carmichael

OTHER BOOKS BY EVELYN CARMICHAEL

Evelyn is the author of the Essential Handbook Series.

Her titles include the following:

<u>Healthy Diet Plans for Health Issues:</u>

<u>The Essential Handbook to Carb Cycling and the Ketogenic Diet</u>

<u>The Essential Handbook to Lectin</u>

<u>The Essential Handbook to a Healthy Gut</u>

<u>The Essential Handbook to the Anti-Inflammation Diet</u>

<u>The Essential Handbook to the High Fiber Diet</u>

<u>The Essential Handbook to Reversing Prediabetes and Diabetes: Meal Plans and Recipes to Reduce Your</u>

Evelyn Carmichael

Blood Sugar Levels and Eliminate Diabetes and Prediabetes

The Essential Handbook to the Alzheimer's Diet

The Essential Handbook to Hashimoto's

The Essential Handbook for Choosing the Right Diet: A Guide to the Most Popular Diets and If They are Right for You

Anti-Inflammation and Super Foods:

The Essential Handbook to Avocados: The Superfood that Reduce Inflammation and lowers blood sugar, blood pressure, and your cholesterol

The Essential Handbook to Turmeric and Ginger: The Anti-Inflammatory Duo that will Change your Life

The Essential Handbook to Coconut Oil: Tips, Recipes, and How to use for weight loss and in your daily life

The Essential Handbook to Apple Cider Vinegar: Tips and Recipes for Weight Loss and Improving your Health, Beauty, & Home

The Essential Handbook to Intermittent Fasting

The Essential Handbook to Superfood Smoothies

Instant Pot Cookbooks:

The Essential Handbook to Low Lectin Instant Pot Cooking

The Essential Handbook to Diabetic Instant Pot Cooking

The Essential Handbook to Paleo Instant Pot Cooking

The Essential Handbook to Gluten Free Instant Pot Cooking

Healthy Living:

The Essential Handbook to Essential Oils: Tips and Recipes for Weight Loss, Stress Relief, and Pain Management

The Essential Handbook to Hygge

The Art of Keeping Goals

AUTHOR NOTE

If you enjoyed this book, found it useful or otherwise then I'd really appreciate it if you would post a short review on Amazon. I do read all the reviews personally so that I can continually write what people are wanting.

Thanks for your support!